Title: The ABC's of Strength and Endurance

The Essential Handbook for Strength and Endurance Success

Introduction:

In the pursuit of a healthier, fitter, and more resilient lifestyle, it's essential to understand that strength and endurance are not just physical attributes but also qualities that encompass mental and emotional fortitude. "The ABC's of Strength and Endurance" is a comprehensive guide that takes you through an alphabetical journey, exploring words and concepts that contribute to your overall well-being and vitality. Each chapter delves into a unique aspect of building and maintaining strength and endurance, offering insights, tips, and practical advice to help you achieve your fitness goals.

Chapter 1: Attitude - The Cornerstone of Strength and Endurance

Developing a positive attitude lays the foundation for your journey toward strength and endurance. Learn how to cultivate a mindset that empowers you to overcome challenges and stay committed.

Your journey toward building strength and endurance begins not with the weights you lift or the miles you run, but with a fundamental aspect of yourself: your attitude. The power of attitude cannot be overstated; it shapes your outlook, influences your decisions, and determines your resilience in the face of challenges. In this chapter, we delve into the profound impact of a positive attitude on your pursuit of physical and mental fortitude.

The Attitude Advantage:

Imagine your attitude as the compass guiding you through uncharted territories. A positive attitude becomes the wind beneath your wings, propelling you forward even when the road gets tough. It's the driving force that transforms obstacles into stepping stones and setbacks into opportunities for growth.

Cultivating a Positive Mindset:

Awareness: Begin by recognizing your current mindset. Are you prone to self-doubt and negativity, or do you approach challenges with a sense of possibility? Awareness is the first step toward transformation.

Mindful Self-Talk: Pay attention to your inner dialogue. Replace self-limiting beliefs with empowering affirmations. Instead of "I can't do it," embrace "I am capable of overcoming any obstacle."

Gratitude Practice: Incorporate a daily gratitude practice to shift your focus from what you lack to what you have accomplished. Gratitude nurtures a positive perspective.

Visualization: Envision yourself succeeding in your fitness endeavors. Visualization not only boosts confidence but also prepares your mind for the journey ahead.

The Resilience Connection:

A positive attitude and resilience go hand in hand. When challenges arise, your attitude determines whether you crumble or rise. Embracing setbacks as temporary and surmountable fosters the resilience needed to persist.

Overcoming Obstacles:

Mind Over Matter: Approach challenges with a "can-do" attitude. Believe that your mind has the power to influence your body's capabilities.

Reframing Challenges: Rather than viewing obstacles as roadblocks, see them as opportunities for growth. Each challenge conquered adds to your strength and endurance.

Staying Committed: A positive attitude fuels your commitment. When enthusiasm wanes, your attitude keeps the fire burning, propelling you forward even when motivation dwindles.

Building a Supportive Environment:

Your attitude doesn't exist in isolation; it's influenced by your surroundings. Surround yourself with individuals who uplift, motivate, and believe in your journey. A supportive community reinforces your positive attitude and helps you stay the course.

Incorporating Attitude into Training:

Mindful Movement: Infuse your workouts with positive intention. Approach each exercise with focus and determination, and let the joy of movement energize you.

Embracing Challenges: Seek out new challenges to test your attitude. Whether it's a longer run, a heavier weight, or a new fitness discipline, approach it with eagerness.

Reflect and Adjust: Regularly assess your attitude and its impact on your progress. If negativity creeps in, acknowledge it and make conscious efforts to reframe your thoughts.

Conclusion:

Your attitude is a beacon that guides you through the highs and lows of your journey toward strength and endurance. It empowers you to rise above challenges, celebrate victories, and stay committed even when the path seems steep. Cultivating a positive attitude is a skill that can be honed, and with practice, it becomes the bedrock upon which you build your physical and mental fortitude. As you move forward, remember that your attitude shapes not only your journey but the very essence of who you become along the way.

Chapter 2: Balance

Discover the importance of balance in your physical activities, nutrition, and daily life. Find harmony between strength-building exercises and recovery, as well as maintaining equilibrium in your diet.

Chapter 2: Balance - Harmonizing Strength, Recovery, and Nutrition

Balance is the art of finding equilibrium in all aspects of your journey toward strength and endurance. Just as a tightrope walker maintains stability, you too must find your balance between exertion and restoration, between building strength and allowing recovery, and between nourishing your body and indulging in moderation. In this chapter, we explore the profound significance of balance and how it contributes to your overall well-being.

The Balance Equation:

Picture balance as the delicate dance between pushing your limits and respecting your boundaries. It involves listening to your body's cues and responding with mindfulness. Achieving balance requires intention, awareness, and a willingness to adapt.

Physical Balance:

Strength Training and Recovery: Recognize that gains are made not during the workout, but in the recovery that follows. Allow time for your muscles to repair and grow stronger after intense strength sessions.

Cross-Training: Incorporate a variety of exercises to prevent overuse injuries and to target different muscle groups. Balance high-intensity workouts with lower-impact activities like yoga or swimming.

Rest and Active Recovery: Prioritize quality sleep to aid recovery. Embrace active recovery methods such as stretching, foam rolling, or light cardio to keep your body supple and ready for your next challenge.

Nutritional Balance:

Nutrient-Dense Diet: Fuel your body with a balanced mix of macronutrients (proteins, carbohydrates, and fats) and micronutrients (vitamins and minerals). Emphasize whole, unprocessed foods.

Portion Control: Practice portion awareness to avoid overeating. Mindful eating allows you to savor your meals and recognize when you're satiated.

Indulgence in Moderation: While it's important to nourish your body, occasional treats can be enjoyed guilt-free. Balance healthier choices with occasional indulgences.

Daily Life Balance:

Time Management: Allocate time for workouts, rest, work, and leisure. Strive for a balance between your fitness goals and other responsibilities.

Stress Management: Find outlets to manage stress, such as meditation, journaling, or spending time in nature. Stress can disrupt balance, so nurturing your mental well-being is crucial.

Social and Personal Life: Dedicate time to relationships and activities that bring joy and fulfillment. Balancing personal and social needs contributes to a well-rounded life.

Applying Balance in Practice:

Personalized Approach: Recognize that balance varies from person to person. Listen to your body's signals and adjust your approach accordingly.

Progressive Overload: Gradually increase the intensity of your workouts to avoid burnout. Balance challenging sessions with easier ones to prevent plateauing and reduce the risk of injury.

Nutrient Timing: Consider when you consume nutrients to optimize performance and recovery. Proper timing of meals and snacks can enhance your energy levels.

Conclusion:

Balance is not a static state but a dynamic process that evolves as you progress in your strength and endurance journey. Finding equilibrium between pushing your limits and respecting your body's needs is the cornerstone of sustainable growth. Embrace the yin and yang of your physical activities, nutrition, and daily life, and you'll create a harmonious path toward enhanced strength, endurance, and overall well-being. Just as a symphony relies on the balance of different instruments, your journey to a healthier you relies on the orchestration of various elements in harmony.

Chapter 3: Consistency

Consistency is key to progress. Explore strategies for establishing consistent workout routines, dietary habits, and mental practices that contribute to long-term success.

Chapter 3: Consistency - The Steady Path to Long-Term Success

In the pursuit of strength and endurance consistency emerges as the guiding light that illuminates your path to progress. The power of consistency lies in its ability to transform short-term efforts into sustainable, long-term achievements. In this chapter, we delve into the importance of consistency and discover strategies to establish unwavering workout routines, dietary habits, and mental practices.

The Consistency Effect:

Consistency lays the foundation for building habits that fortify your physical and mental well-being. When you commit to regular actions, whether in exercise, nutrition, or mindfu ness, you create a positive ripple effect that transcends individual moments and leads to transformative results.

Establishing a Consistent Workout Routine:

Set Realistic Goals: Define clear, achievable goals for your fitness journey. Break them down into smaller milestones to track your progress effectively.

Create a Schedule: Plan your workouts in advance, integrating them into your daily or weekly calendar. Treating exercise as an essential appointment helps prioritize its consistency.

Find Your Ideal Time: Discover the time of day that suits your energy levels and schedule best for exercise. Whether it's morning, afternoon, or evening, consistency thrives when your workouts align with your natural rhythm.

Variety with Structure: While embracing variety is essential, maintaining some structure in your routine ensures consistency. Designate specific days for strength training, cardio, and recovery.

Nurturing Consistent Dietary Habits:

Meal Prepping: Prepare healthy meals and snacks in advance to avoid making impulsive choices when hungry. Having nutritious options readily available supports dietary consistency.

Mindful Eating: Practice mindful eating to savor your meals and recognize when you're satisfied. Slow down, listen to your body's hunger and fullness cues, and avoid distractions while eating.

Hydration: Stay consistent with your water intake throughout the day. Hydration is key to maintaining energy levels and supporting your body's functions.

Indulgence in Moderation: While consistency is vital, allow yourself occasional treats without guilt. Embrace balance and remember that a single indulgence won't derail your overall progress.

Cultivating Consistency in Mental Practices:

Mindfulness Meditation: Dedicate time to mindfulness meditation to nurture a calmer, focused mind. Consistent meditation helps manage stress and enhances mental resilience.

Positive Affirmations: Integrate positive affirmations into your daily routine to reinforce a growth mindset. Consistently affirming your capabilities bolsters confidence.

Journaling: Maintain a journal to track your progress, reflect on challenges and victories, and gain insights into your journey. Consistent journaling fosters self-awareness.

Visualization: Regularly visualize yourself succeeding in your fitness endeavors. Consistency in visualization enhances mental preparation for upcoming challenges.

Overcoming Obstacles to Consistency:

Accountability Partners: Seek accountability partners or join fitness communities to stay motivated and committed. Sharing your journey with others provides encouragement.

Adaptability: Life is dynamic, and obstacles may arise. Embrace adaptability and adjust your approach when necessary, while remaining steadfast in your commitment.

Celebrate Small Wins: Recognize and celebrate each small victory on your journey. Consistent acknowledgment of progress fuels motivation.

Conclusion:

Consistency isn't about perfection but rather about a continuous commitment to improvement. By establishing consistent workout routines, dietary habits, and mental practices, you cultivate the resilience needed to overcome challenges and achieve long-term success in your pursuit of strength and endurance. Embrace the power of consistency as a compass guiding you toward a healthier, fitter, and more enduring version of yourself. In the symphony of your fitness journey, consistency provides the rhythm that harmonizes your actions, leading to transformative melodies of growth and achievement.

Chapter 4: Determination

Uncover the strength that comes from unwavering determination. Learn how setting and working toward achievable goals fuels your endurance journey.

Chapter 4: Determination - Igniting Endurance through Unwavering Purpose

In the realm of strength and endurance, determination stands as the bedrock of success, the driving force that propels you forward, unwavering, in the face of challenges. It's the fierce commitment that transforms dreams into reality and turns aspirations into achievements. In this chapter, we delve into the profound power of determination and its role in fuelling your journey of endurance.

The Essence of Determination:

Determination is the heartbeat of your endurance journey. It's the inner fire that refuses to be extinguished by setbacks, doubts, or obstacles. It's not mere stubbornness; rather, it's the unwavering belief that your goals are within reach, and the unyielding dedication to making them a reality.

Setting and Pursuing Achievable Goals:

The North Star: Goals serve as your compass, guiding you toward a destination. Set clear, specific, and achievable objectives that align with your endurance aspirations. Visualize where you want to go, and let determination chart the course.

Break it Down: Complex goals can be overwhelming. Break them into smaller, manageable steps. Each achievement becomes a stepping stone, strengthening your determination with every step forward.

The Power of Progress: The journey is as important as the destination. Measure your progress to acknowledge how far you've come. Each milestone reached is a testament to your determination and provides renewed motivation.

Cultivating Determination:

Purposeful Passion: Connect your goals to a deeper purpose. Understand why you're embarking on this journey of endurance. When your goals are infused with meaning, determination thrives.

Positive Affirmations: Consistently reaffirm your determination through positive self-talk. Replace self-doubt with affirmations that bolster your confidence and keep your determination burning bright.

Resilience and Adaptability: Determination doesn't eliminate challenges; it equips you to face them head-on. Embrace setbacks as lessons, not defeats. Let them fuel your determination to overcome and adapt.

Drawing Strength from Determination:

Mental Resilience: Determination is the shield against doubt and adversity. When challenges arise, remind yourself of your unwavering commitment, using it as a source of inner strength.

Motivation Booster: Motivation can ebb and flow, but determination persists. Even on days when motivation wanes, your determination keeps you moving forward.

Inspirational Examples: Study stories of individuals who demonstrated remarkable determination. Their journeys of triumph over adversity can fuel your own determination.

Embracing the Journey:

Celebrating Victories: Each achievement, no matter how small, is a testament to your determination. Celebrate these wins as a reminder of your capability to overcome obstacles.

Mindful Reflection: Regularly reflect on your journey. Note the challenges you've conquered, the progress you've made, and the determination that's led you this far.

Fueling the Flame: Surround yourself with positive influences, supportive communities, and inspiration that stokes your determination. The collective energy of these elements bolsters your resolve.

Conclusion:

Determination is the heartbeat of your endurance journey, the energy that keeps you moving when the road gets tough. It's the promise you make to yourself to stay the course, even when challenges arise. By setting achievable goals and nurturing unwavering determination, you are not only building endurance but also fostering a mindset of resilience, growth, and unyielding strength. Remember, determination is not a fleeting emotion; it's a conscious choice to embrace the challenges and opportunities that shape your journey.

Chapter 5: Empowerment

Empower yourself with knowledge and self-awareness. Understand your body's limits and capabilities, and harness the mental strength needed to push through barriers.

Chapter 5: Empowerment - Embracing Knowledge and Mental Fortitude

In the realm of strength and endurance, empowerment is the crown jewel that adorns your journey. It is the harmonious marriage of knowledge, self-awareness, and mental strength that enables you to transcend limits and unleash your full potential. In this chapter, we explore the transformative power of empowerment and how it shapes your understanding of your body's capabilities and the fortitude needed to overcome barriers.

The Foundation of Empowerment:

Empowerment begins with knowledge, for knowledge is the key that unlocks the mysteries of your body and its boundless potential. It is the understanding of how your muscles work, how your energy systems function, and how your body adapts to training stimuli. Knowledge, combined with self-awareness, is the fue that ignites the fire of empowerment.

Understanding Your Body:

Body Awareness: Tune in to your body's signals and cues during workouts. Recognize when you need to push harder and when to allow for rest and recovery.

Physical Limits and Progression: Empowerment comes from understanding that your body has limits, but those limits can expand with consistent, progressive training. Embrace the journey of growth and improvement.

Rest and Recovery: Appreciate the importance of rest and recovery in your fitness journey. Understand that recovery is not a sign of weakness but a crucial aspect of achieving optimal performance.

The Mental Fortitude:

Self-Belief: Empowerment is grounded in unwavering self-belief. Cultivate a positive mindset that reminds you of your strength and potential, even in the face of challenges.

Overcoming Barriers: Empowerment is not about eliminating obstacles but embracing them as opportunities for growth. Develop mental resilience to tackle barriers head-on.

Visualization and Goal-Setting: Visualize yourself achieving your goals. Set clear, meaningful objectives and use visualization as a tool to bolster your mental strength.

Empowering with Knowledge:

Educate Yourself: Continuously seek knowledge about exercise, nutrition, and recovery. Understanding the science behind your fitness routine empowers you to make informed decisions.

Seek Professional Guidance: Consult with fitness experts or coaches to receive personalized guidance. Their expertise will help you progress safely and efficiently.

Listen to Your Body: Empowerment comes from respecting and honoring your body's needs. Learn to distinguish between discomfort that leads to growth and pain that requires attention.

Embracing Challenges and Growth:

Stepping out of Comfort Zones: Empowerment arises when you dare to step beyond your comfort zone. Embrace challenges that push you to new heights.

Learn from Setbacks: Empowerment is not deterred by setbacks but motivated by the lessons they impart. View setbacks as stepping stones to future success.

Celebrating Achievements: Acknowledge and celebrate your achievements, both big and small. Recognizing progress fuels empowerment and motivates you to push further.

Conclusion:

Empowerment is the beacon that illuminates your path of strength and endurance. By combining knowledge and self-awareness with mental fortitude, you create a force that transcends physical barriers and propels you toward greatness. Embrace the transformative power of empowerment as you understand your body, believe in your capabilities, and harness the knowledge and mental strength needed to push through challenges. Remember, empowerment is not a destination; it's a lifelong journey of self-discovery and growth, and it holds the key to unlocking the limitless potential within you.

Chapter 6: Flexibility

Flexibility is a cornerstone of endurance. Discover the benefits of maintaining a flexible body and mind and how it contributes to overall strength.

Chapter 6: Flexibility - Nurturing Body and Mind for Endurance Excellence

In the realm of strength and endurance, flexibility stands as a vital pillar that supports your journey toward greatness. It extends beyond the physical, weaving a harmonious tapestry of suppleness between body and mind. In this chapter, we delve into the profound significance of flexibility, exploring how its presence enriches your endurance pursuits and contributes to the cultivation of overall strength.

The Essence of Flexibility:

Flexibility transcends the realm of mere physical contortion; it embodies adaptability, resilience, and the willingness to embrace change. Just as a supple body can move through various ranges of motion, a flexible mind can navigate the twists and turns of challenges with grace.

Physical Flexibility:

Enhanced Range of Motion: A flexible body exhibits increased joint mobility and muscle elasticity, which directly translates to improved performance in endurance activities. Each movement becomes more fluid and efficient.

Injury Prevention: Supple muscles and joints are less prone to injury. Flexibility ensures that your body can withstand the demands of training without succumbing to strains or overuse injuries.

Post-Workout Recovery: Incorporating flexibility exercises into your routine aids in post-workout recovery. Stretching soothes tired muscles, reduces muscle soreness, and promotes relaxation.

Mental Flexibility:

Adaptability: A flexible mind can adapt to changing circumstances and navigate unexpected challenges. Developing mental flexibility allows you to adjust your strategies and stay resilient in the face of setbacks.

Open-Mindedness: Embracing new training techniques, nutritional approaches, or mental practices requires an open mind. Mental flexibility enables you to explore different avenues to enhance your endurance journey.

Stress Management: A flexible mind can better manage stress and anxiety. By cultivating mental flexibility, you can approach stressors with a calmer perspective and develop effective coping strategies.

Balancing Act - Body and Mind:

Stretching Routine: Integrate regular stretching sessions into your routine. Dynamic stretches before workouts prepare your body for movement, while static stretches afterward promote muscle recovery and flexibility.

Mindfulness and Meditation: Practice mindfulness and meditation to cultivate mental flexibility. These techniques enhance your ability to embrace the present moment and adapt to changing circumstances.

Yoga and Pilates: Engage in yoga or Pilates sessions, both of which emphasize flexibility of both body and mind. These disciplines foster balance, strength, and mental clarity.

The Fusion of Strength and Flexibility:

Synergistic Relationship: Flexibility and strength are not opposing forces but symbiotic partners. A strong, flexible body is less prone to injury and capable of achieving optimal performance.

Endurance Benefits: Combining strength and flexibility amplifies endurance capabilities. A flexible body expends less energy during movement, resulting in increased stamina and improved efficiency.

Mind-Body Harmony: The fusion of strength and flexibility creates a harmonious unity between body and mind. This synergy fosters a holistic sense of well-being and empowers you to conquer endurance challenges with unwavering confidence.

Conclusion:

Flexibility is not a trait reserved for the gymnast or the yogi; it's a cornerstone of endurance excellence that embraces both body and mind.

By nurturing physical flexibility, you grant your body the freedom to move with grace and efficiency, minimizing the risk of injury and enhancing your endurance capabilities. Simultaneously, cultivating mental flexibility empowers you to adapt, innovate, and thrive in the face of challenges. Remember, flexibility is not a sign of weakness; it's an emblem of strength that unites body and mind in a symphony of movement, resilience, and enduring success.

Chapter 7: Gratitude

Cultivate gratitude for your body's capabilities and the opportunities to enhance your strength and endurance. Explore the link between gratitude and mental resilience.

Chapter 7: Gratitude - Nurturing Resilience through Appreciation

In the realm of strength and endurance, gratitude emerges as a powerful elixir, enriching your journey with profound significance. It transforms mere physical pursuits into heartfelt endeavors, connecting you to the profound privilege of enhancing your strength and endurance. In this chapter, we embark on a journey of exploration, unveiling the transformative link between gratitude, mental resilience, and the boundless potential that lies within.

The Essence of Gratitude:

Gratitude is not a mere platitude; it is a dynamic force that elevates your endurance journey to new heights. It is the act of acknowledging and cherishing the capabilities of your body, while also recognizing the invaluable opportunities for growth that lie before you.

Gratitude and Body Appreciation:

Honoring Your Body: Gratitude allows you to celebrate your body's unique capabilities. It's a reminder to treat your body with respect and care, nurturing its strength and agility.

Mindful Movement: Infuse your workouts with gratitude. Engage in each exercise with a sense of appreciation, relishing the intricate mechanics of your body in motion.

Recovery and Self-Care: Gratitude extends to recovery. Treat rest and recovery as acts of self-love, acknowledging the importance of rejuvenation for sustained endurance.

Gratitude's Resilience-Building Power:

Positive Perspective: Cultivating gratitude nurtures a positive mindset. By focusing on what you have, rather than what you lack, you build a foundation of mental resilience that supports you through challenges.

Adversity as Growth: Gratitude reframes adversity as a catalyst for growth. Rather than viewing setbacks as roadblocks, approach them as opportunities to learn, adapt, and emerge stronger.

Stress Alleviation: Gratitude acts as a buffer against stress. When you appreciate the journey and the process, stress loses its grip, and you approach challenges with a clearer, more composed mindset.

Practicing Gratitude:

Daily Reflection: Dedicate time each day to reflect on the aspects of your endurance journey for which you're grateful. These can range from small achievements to the overall journey itself.

Gratitude Journal: Maintain a gratitude journal to record your reflections. Writing down your appreciation reinforces the positive impact gratitude has on your mindset.

Mindful Moments: Infuse your daily routine with moments of gratitude. Whether during warm-ups, cool-downs, or moments of pause, take a breath and express gratitude for your journey.

Gratitude's Ripple Effect:

Empathy and Connection: Gratitude extends beyond yourself, fostering empathy for others on their journeys. As you appreciate your growth, you encourage and support those around you.

Endurance with Purpose: Infusing your journey with gratitude infuses it with purpose. It's no longer just about building strength; it's about embracing each step with thankfulness and intention.

Sustaining Motivation: Gratitude fuels intrinsic motivation. It reminds you why you started your endurance journey and helps you stay committed, even when external motivation wanes.

Conclusion:

Gratitude is the thread that weaves the fabric of your endurance journey, connecting every stride, lift, and stretch with a sense of purpose and appreciation. As you cultivate gratitude for your body's capabilities and the opportunities to enhance your strength and endurance, you forge a resilient mindset that navigates challenges with grace. Embrace gratitude not as a fleeting emotion, but as an enduring companion that guides you through the highs and lows of your journey. Remember, gratitude is not just a feeling; it's a state of being that propels you toward mental resilience, profound self-discovery, and enduring fulfillment.

Chapter 8: Hydration

Hydration is essential for endurance. Learn about the role of water in maintaining energy levels and optimizing physical performance.

Chapter 8: Hydration - The Elixir of Endurance

In the realm of strength and endurance, hydration stands as the life-giving elixir that fuels your journey towards greatness. Water, a seemingly simple and abundant resource, plays a profound role in maintaining energy levels, optimizing physical performance, and ensuring you reach the pinnacle of your endurance pursuits. In this chapter, we unveil the crucial significance of hydration and how it acts as the essential pillar of success in your endurance journey.

The Essence of Hydration:

Hydration is more than just quenching your thirst; it's a fundamental element that governs your body's ability to function optimally. When you're well-hydrated, your body can efficiently perform tasks, recover from training, and adapt to challenges.

The Role of Water in Endurance:

Maintaining Energy Levels: Water is the conduit through which nutrients and energy are transported to your muscles during endurance activities. Proper hydration ensures that your body can maintain energy levels and sustain performance.

Thermoregulation: During exercise, your body generates heat. Sweating is a natural cooling mechanism, but it requires an adequate supply of water. Proper hydration enables effective thermoregulation, preventing overheating and heat-related illnesses.

Muscle Function and Recovery: Dehydration can lead to muscle cramps and impair muscle function. Sufficient water intake aids in muscle contraction, recovery, and overall performance.

The Importance of Fluid Balance:

Preventing Dehydration: Dehydration adversely impacts endurance. It reduces blood volume, making your heart work harder to pump oxygen and nutrients to muscles. This can lead to premature fatigue and reduced performance.

Avoiding Overhydration: While staying hydrated is essential, overhydration can be equally harmful. Overconsumption of water can lead to a condition called hyponatremia, where sodium levels in the blood become dangerously low.

Individual Hydration Needs: Hydration requirements vary from person to person, based on factors such as body weight, activity level, and environmental conditions. Listen to your body's cues and adjust your hydration accordingly.

Hydration Strategies for Endurance:

Pre-Exercise Hydration: Begin your endurance activity well-hydrated. Drink water in the hours leading up to your workout to ensure your body starts with adequate fluid levels.

During Exercise Hydration: During prolonged endurance activities, aim to consume water regularly. Sip water at regular intervals, and consider using sports drinks to replenish electrolytes lost through sweat.

Post-Exercise Hydration: After your workout, continue hydrating to replenish the fluid lost during exercise. Opt for water, and consider incorporating hydrating foods like fruits and vegetables into your post-workout meal.

Staying Mindful of Hydration:

Thirst as a Guide: Pay attention to your thirst cues. Thirst is your body's way of signaling that it needs water, so don't ignore it.

Monitoring Hydration Levels: Check the color of your urine to gauge your hydration status. Light-colored urine generally indicates adequate hydration, while dark-colored urine suggests dehydration.

Hydration and Everyday Habits: Hydration isn't limited to workouts; it's a daily commitment. Cultivate a habit of drinking water throughout the day to maintain optimal hydration levels.

Conclusion:

Hydration is the unsung hero that breathes life into your endurance journey. By understanding the role of water in maintaining energy levels, optimizing physical performance, and promoting overall well-being, you elevate your endurance pursuits to new heights. Embrace hydration not as a mere necessity but as a powerful ally that empowers your body to conquer challenges and achieve greatness. Remember, the key to endurance excellence lies in the simple act of staying hydrated, unlocking the boundless potential that awaits you on this transformative journey.

Chapter 9: Intensity

Explore the right balance of intensity in your workouts. Understand how varying levels of intensity contribute to strength and endurance gains.

Chapter 9: Intensity - The Art of Balanced Progress

In the realm of strength and endurance, intensity emerges as both a guide and a challenge, a dynamic force that propels you forward on your journey to greatness. It is the delicate dance between pushing your limits and honoring your body's needs, a nuanced art that dictates the pace of your progress. In this chapter, we delve into the multifaceted nature of intensity, uncovering its role in sculpting strength and endurance gains and deciphering the intricate balance required to harness its power.

The Essence of Intensity:

Intensity is the driving force behind transformative change. It is the spark that ignites growth, pushing your body beyond its comfort zone and compelling it to adapt and evolve. When wielded wisely, intensity becomes the catalyst for strength and endurance gains that redefine your limits.

Understanding Intensity and Progress:

Gradual Progression: Intensity should be a gradual journey. Start with manageable levels and progressively increase it over time to prevent overexertion and reduce the risk of injury.

Targeting Different Energy Systems: Varying levels of intensity engage different energy systems in your body. Low-intensity workouts tap into aerobic endurance, while high-intensity intervals activate anaerobic systems, fostering a holistic approach to strength and endurance gains.

Balancing Volume and Intensity: Striking a balance between workout volume (total work) and intensity (effort level) is key. Adjusting this balance based on your goals and recovery capacity ensures sustainable progress.

Intensity's Role in Strength Gains:

Muscle Fiber Recruitment: Higher intensity workouts recruit a greater number of muscle fibers, leading to enhanced muscle growth and strength development.

Progressive Overload: Intensity drives progressive overload, a foundational principle for strength gains. As your body adapts to increased intensity, you continually challenge it to improve.

Neuromuscular Adaptations: Intense workouts improve neuromuscular coordination, enabling your muscles to work more efficiently and generate greater force.

Intensity's Impact on Endurance:

Enhanced Cardiovascular Fitness: High-intensity interval training (HIIT) and other intense endurance workouts improve cardiovascular fitness by pushing your heart and lungs to adapt and become more efficient.

Lactic Acid Threshold: Intense workouts elevate your lactic acid threshold, allowing you to sustain higher levels of effort before fatigue sets in.

Efficient Energy Utilization: Mixing high and low-intensity workouts teaches your body to switch between energy sources, optimizing energy utilization during endurance activities.

Personalizing Intensity for Success:

Goals and Progress Markers: Align intensity levels with your goals. Whether you aim for strength, endurance, or a blend of both, tailor your workouts accordingly.

Listen to Your Body: Prioritize your body's signals. Push yourself, but not to the point of burnout. Strive for challenge, not recklessness.

Periodization: Implement periodization in your training plan. Cycle through phases of low, moderate, and high intensity to prevent plateaus and promote continuous progress.

Embracing the Intensity Journey:

Mindful Preparation: Mentally prepare for intense workouts. Set clear intentions and embrace the challenge with a positive mindset.

Recovery and Rest: Intense workouts require adequate recovery. Prioritize sleep, nutrition, and active recovery methods to optimize your body's response to intensity.

Celebrating Small Wins: Acknowledge and celebrate progress. Each step forward, no matter how small, is a testament to your dedication and the intelligent use of intensity.

Conclusion:

Intensity is a potent tool, a double-edged sword that can elevate your strength and endurance to extraordinary heights when harnessed with precision. By understanding the nuanced interplay of intensity levels, you sculpt a journey that leads to consistent progress and surpasses your boundaries. Approach intensity as an ally, not an adversary, and let it guide you towards your aspirations. Remember, in the art of balanced progress, intensity is the brushstroke that paints the masterpiece of your strength and endurance gains.

Chapter 10: Joy

Find joy in the process of improving your strength and endurance. Discover how incorporating activities you love enhances your overall well-being.

Chapter 10: Joy - Fueling the Endurance Journey

In the realm of strength and endurance, joy stands as the radiant sun that illuminates your path to greatness. It is the contagious energy that infuses every step of your journey with enthusiasm and purpose. In this chapter, we dive into the transformative power of joy, exploring how finding delight in the process of improvement, and incorporating activities you love, enhances not only your physical performance but also your overall well-being.

The Essence of Joy:

Joy is the heart of your endurance journey, the essence that makes each moment count. It transcends the sweat and effort, transforming mere workouts into exhilarating experiences that nourish your body, mind, and soul.

Joy and Physical Performance:

Effort as Fun: When you find joy in the process, effort becomes an enjoyable challenge rather than a burden. You approach workouts with a playful spirit, which enhances your performance.

Endorphin Release: Joy triggers the release of endorphins, your body's natural mood enhancers. This surge of positive chemicals not only elevates your mood but also reduces stress and pain perception.

Consistency and Dedication: Joy fosters consistency in your training. When you engage in activities you love, you are more likely to remain dedicated to your endurance journey.

The Power of Activities You Love:

Intrinsic Motivation: Engaging in activities you love taps into intrinsic motivation. You are driven by the sheer joy of doing what you enjoy, rather than external rewards.

Flow State: Activities that bring you joy often lead to the flow state, where you are fully immersed and completely absorbed in the present moment. This state of heightened focus enhances your performance.

Balancing Challenge and Skill: Joyful activities strike the perfect balance between challenge and skill level. They challenge you enough to keep you engaged while leveraging your existing abilities.

Enhancing Well-Being:

Stress Reduction: Joy is a natural stress reducer. Engaging in activities that bring you joy helps alleviate stress, promoting overall well-being and mental clarity.

Positive Outlook: Joy cultivates a positive outlook on life. It shapes how you perceive challenges and setbacks, enabling you to maintain resilience and a growth mindset.

Self-Care and Balance: Prioritizing activities you love is an act of self-care. It allows you to strike a balance between your endurance pursuits and other aspects of life.

Finding Joy in the Journey:

Explore New Activities: Be open to trying new activities and sports. You might discover unexpected sources of joy that expand your endurance horizons.

Create Meaningful Connections: Engage in endurance activities with like-minded individuals. Sharing experiences and accomplishments fosters a sense of community and joy.

Celebrate Progress and Achievements: Celebrate every milestone and improvement along your journey. Acknowledging your growth reinforces the joy of progress.

Embracing Joy as a Foundation:

Mindful Presence: Embrace the present moment with mindful awareness. Find joy in the sensations, the movements, and the unfolding of your endurance pursuits.

Playfulness and Fun: Infuse playfulness and fun into your workouts. It could be dancing to your favorite music, adding playful challenges, or exploring new routes.

Embodying Gratitude: Cultivate gratitude for the joy that accompanies your endurance journey. Let it fuel your passion and appreciation for every opportunity to improve and grow.

Conclusion:

Joy is the luminous thread that weaves the fabric of your endurance journey. By finding delight in the process of improvement and incorporating activities you love, you unlock a wellspring of vitality that infuses your every endeavor. Embrace joy not as a fleeting emotion but as an enduring source of inspiration that nourishes your body, enriches your mind, and uplifts your soul. Remember, joy is not a destination; it is a cherished companion that accompanies you on the transformative and joyous path to strength, endurance, and a life lived to the fullest.

Chapter 11: Knowledge

Educate yourself about proper training techniques, nutrition, and recovery strategies. Knowledge empowers you to make informed decisions for your fitness journey.

Chapter 11: Knowledge - The Empowerment of Informed Endurance

In the realm of strength and endurance, knowledge stands as the guiding compass, illuminating your path to optimal performance and well-being. It is the foundation upon which you build your fitness journey, empowering you to make informed decisions that shape your path to greatness. In this chapter, we delve into the transformative power of knowledge, exploring how educating yourself about proper training techniques, nutrition, and recovery strategies elevates your endurance pursuits to new heights.

The Essence of Knowledge:

Knowledge is the cornerstone of your endurance journey. It is the arsenal of information that equips you with the tools to navigate challenges, make wise choices, and unlock your full potential.

The Importance of Proper Training Techniques:

Efficiency and Effectiveness: Knowledge of proper training techniques ensures your workouts are efficient and effective, maximizing the benefits of your efforts.

Injury Prevention: Understanding correct form and technique reduces the risk of injuries during endurance activities, safeguarding your body and promoting longevity.

Progressive Training: Knowledge allows you to structure progressive training plans that challenge your body while allowing for adequate recovery and adaptation.

The Power of Nutrition:

Fueling Performance: Educating yourself about nutrition equips you to provide your body with the necessary fuel to perform at its best during endurance activities.

Recovery and Repair: Proper nutrition supports the recovery and repair of muscles after intense workouts, enhancing your body's ability to adapt and grow stronger.

Sustainable Eating Habits: Knowledge empowers you to develop sustainable and balanced eating habits, promoting overall health and well-being beyond your endurance pursuits.

Recovery Strategies for Optimal Performance:

Understanding Rest: Knowledge of recovery strategies helps you appreciate the importance of rest in the overall training process. Rest allows your body to rebuild and rejuvenate.

Active Recovery: Knowledge of active recovery techniques, such as stretching and light exercises, aids in reducing muscle soreness and enhancing flexibility.

Sleep Optimization: Educating yourself about the significance of quality sleep fosters better sleep habits, ensuring your body receives the restorative rest it needs.

Empowering Informed Decisions:

Learning from Experts: Seek guidance from experienced coaches, trainers, or professionals who can impart valuable knowledge and expertise.

Research and Reading: Stay curious and read extensively about endurance training, nutrition, and recovery. Arm yourself with evidence-based information.

Trial and Reflection: Experiment with different training techniques, nutrition plans, and recovery strategies. Reflect on how each approach impacts your performance and well-being.

Knowledge for Lifelong Endurance:

Continuous Learning: Embrace a mindset of continuous learning. The world of endurance training is constantly evolving, and staying informed ensures you remain at the forefront.

Teaching Others: Share your knowledge with fellow enthusiasts. Teaching others solidifies your understanding while also empowering them on their own journeys.

Adapting to Change: Be open to new ideas and adapt your approach as you gain knowledge. Embrace change as a pathway to growth and improvement.

Conclusion:

Knowledge is the empowering force that breathes life into your endurance journey. By educating yourself about proper training techniques, nutrition, and recovery strategies, you build a resilient foundation for success. Armed with knowledge, you transcend the limitations of the unknown, embrace informed decisions, and unlock the full potential of your body and mind. Remember, knowledge is the bridge that connects aspiration with achievement, transforming your endurance pursuit into a transformative and lifelong journey of strength, performance, and well-being.

Chapter 12: Limits

Recognize and challenge your limits to continuously grow in strength and endurance. Understand when to push yourself and when to respect your boundaries.

Chapter 12: Limits - Breaking Barriers and Embracing Boundaries

In the realm of strength and endurance, limits stand as the thresholds that beckon both exploration and reverence. They are the frontiers of possibility, urging you to challenge and expand them while also reminding you to embrace the wisdom of restraint. In this chapter, we delve into the complex interplay of limits, exploring how recognizing and challenging them enables continuous growth in strength and endurance, and understanding when to push yourself and when to respect your boundaries becomes the guiding compass of your journey.

The Essence of Limits:

Limits are not constraints but invitations to push the boundaries of your potential. They are the signposts that guide your progress and protect you from overexertion. Understanding limits allows you to cultivate a balanced and sustainable approach to your endurance pursuits.

Challenging Your Limits:

Incremental Progression: Growth lies in gradual and progressive challenges. Set realistic goals and consistently work towards surpassing them, allowing your body to adapt and thrive.

Mind Over Matter: The mind often dictates the body's capabilities. Recognize self-imposed mental limits and break through them to unleash untapped reservoirs of strength and endurance.

Surpassing Comfort Zones: Endurance gains are often found beyond the comfort of familiarity. Embrace discomfort and uncertainty, for it is in those moments that true growth emerges.

Knowing When to Push:

Distinguishing Discomfort from Pain: Learn to differentiate between the discomfort of pushing your limits and the warning signs of injury or overtraining. Respect your body's signals

Trusting Your Preparation: If you have adequately prepared through consistent training and recovery, you can confidently push your limits, knowing you have laid a strong foundation.

Setting the Right Context: Choose appropriate moments to challenge your limits. Races, competitions, or structured training sessions can be opportune times to test your boundaries.

Embracing Boundaries:

Respecting Rest and Recovery: Your body needs time to recover and rebuild after intense efforts. Embrace rest days and prioritize recovery to prevent burnout and injury.

Adapting to Individual Needs: Recognize that each person's limits and response to training may differ. Avoid comparing yourself to others and honor your unique journey.

The Wisdom of Listening: Pay attention to your body's signals. If you feel persistent fatigue, excessive soreness, or emotional burnout, it may be time to respect your boundaries.

The Balance of Growth and Preservation:

Periodization and Structured Training: Incorporate periodization into your training plan, alternating between intense phases and periods of active recovery.

Holistic Approach to Well-Being: Balance your endurance pursuits with self-care practices, such as meditation, yoga, or hobbies, to nourish your mental and emotional well-being.

Embracing Plateaus: Plateaus are an inherent part of progress. Use these periods to reflect, refocus, and recharge before setting new challenges.

A Journey of Endless Exploration:

Embrace the Process: Embrace the journey, not just the destination. Each step, whether it challenges or respects your limits, contributes to your growth.

Celebrate Every Milestone: Celebrate your accomplishments, no matter how big or small. Acknowledge the effort, dedication, and courage that fuel your pursuit.

Revel in the Unknown: Embrace the beauty of the unknown. The journey to push and respect your limits is an adventure of self-discovery and continuous growth.

Conclusion:

Limits are the guardians of your endurance journey, guiding you towards continuous growth and self-awareness. By recognizing when to challenge your boundaries and when to respect them, you cultivate a balanced and sustainable approach to strength and endurance. Embrace limits not as barriers, but as opportunities to expand and refine your abilities. Remember, the boundaries you encounter are gateways to the vast expanse of your potential, calling you to traverse the landscape of endless exploration, resilience, and growth in your quest for strength and endurance.

Chapter 13: Mindfulness

Practice mindfulness to stay present during workouts, nourish your body with mindful eating, and enhance your mental resilience.

Chapter 13: Mindfulness - The Path to Present and Resilient Endurance

In the realm of strength and endurance, mindfulness stands as the gateway to an elevated and purposeful journey. It is the art of being fully present, infusing each moment with focused awareness and intention. In this chapter, we explore the transformative power of mindfulness, understanding how its practice enriches your workouts, nourishes your body with mindful eating, and enhances your mental resilience to conquer the challenges that lie ahead.

The Essence of Mindfulness:

Mindfulness is the art of presence, unifying the body, mind, and spirit in the tapestry of endurance. It is the conscious act of experiencing each movement, each breath, and each taste with a profound sense of awareness.

Mindfulness in Workouts:

Present-Moment Focus: Mindfulness anchors your attention to the present, fostering a deeper connection with your body and the movements it performs during workouts.

Optimal Performance: By staying present and focused, you optimize your performance, honing your technique, and unlocking the flow state where you become one with your activities.

Emotional Regulation: Mindfulness allows you to recognize and manage emotions that arise during workouts, promoting a more balanced and positive experience.

Mindful Eating for Nourishment:

Savoring Each Bite: When eating mindfully, you savor the flavors, textures, and aroma of your food, creating a more gratifying and nourishing experience.

Awareness of Hunger and Fullness: Mindful eating helps you attune to your body's hunger and fullness cues, guiding you to eat in a way that respects your body's needs.

Cultivating Healthy Habits: Mindfulness dissolves mindless eating patterns, fostering healthier relationships with food and promoting better dietary choices.

Mental Resilience through Mindfulness:

Embracing Challenges: Mindfulness enhances your ability to face challenges with equanimity, viewing them as opportunities for growth rather than obstacles.

Managing Stress: Mindfulness-based stress reduction techniques enable you to manage stress more effectively, fostering mental resilience and emotional well-being.

Cultivating a Growth Mindset: By staying present and mindful, you nurture a growth mindset that views setbacks as temporary and possibilities for improvement as boundless.

Practicing Mindfulness:

Meditative Exercises: Incorporate meditation or breathing exercises into your routine to cultivate mindfulness and train your mind to focus.

Body Scan: During workouts, engage in a body scan to tune into each part of your body, checking for tension and ensuring proper form.

Mindful Eating Rituals: Create rituals around mealtime, such as giving thanks or taking a moment to breathe before eating, to bring mindfulness into your nourishment.

Integrating Mindfulness into Everyday Life:

Beyond Workouts and Meals: Extend mindfulness into your daily activities. Embrace each step, each interaction, and each moment as an opportunity for mindful presence.

Nature Immersion: Spend time in nature immersing yourself in its beauty and tranquility, to enhance mindfulness and recharge your mental resilience.

Gratitude Practice: Cultivate a daily gratitude practice, reflecting on the blessings in your life, and fostering a positive outlook that enriches your endurance journey.

Conclusion:

Mindfulness is the heart of your endurance odyssey, guiding you towards a state of heightened awareness and mental resilience. By practicing mindfulness, you infuse each workout with intention, nourish your body with mindful eating, and build the mental strength needed to overcome obstacles. Remember, mindfulness is not a destination, but an ongoing practice that enriches every aspect of your life. Embrace mindfulness as your ever-present ally, guiding you to the path of purposeful and resilient endurance, where each step is a mindful stride towards a life of balance, strength, and inner harmony.

Chapter 14: Nutrition

Explore the vital role of nutrition in building strength and endurance. Learn about balanced eating, nutrient timing, and fueling your body for optimal performance.

Chapter 14: Nutrition - Fueling the Fire of Strength and Endurance

In the realm of strength and endurance, nutrition is the lifeblood that sustains your journey and empowers your body to reach new heights. It is the art of nourishing yourself with purpose and precision, providing the foundation for peak performance and optimal well-being. In this chapter, we delve into the vital role of nutrition, exploring the significance of balanced eating, nutrient timing, and fueling your body for unparalleled strength and endurance.

The Essence of Nutrition:

Nutrition is the cornerstone of your endurance voyage, fueling your body with the sustenance it requires to excel. It is the synergy between food and performance, shaping not only your physical abilities but also your mental fortitude.

The Power of Balanced Eating:

The Nutrient Symphony: Embrace a balanced diet that includes a rich variety of nutrients such as carbohydrates, proteins, fats, vitamins, and minerals. Each plays a unique role in optimizing your performance.

Sustaining Energy Levels: Balanced eating maintains stable energy levels throughout your workouts, enhancing endurance and reducing fatigue.

Supporting Recovery: Nutrient-dense foods aid in muscle recovery, minimizing post-workout soreness, and preparing your body for the next challenge.

Strategic Nutrient Timing:

Pre-Workout Fueling: Prioritize easily digestible carbohydrates before your workouts to provide readily availab e energy.

During-Workout Nourishment: For longer endurance activities, consider consuming carbohydrates or energy gels to sustain energy levels and delay fatigue.

Post-Workout Recovery: Within the first hour after your workout, consume a mix of carbohydrates and proteins to replenish glycogen stores and promote muscle repair.

Fueling for Optimal Performance:

Individualized Approach: Understand that nutrition needs are unique to each person. Experiment with different foods and timing to discover what works best for you.

Hydration Matters: Proper hydration is crucial for endurance performance. Monitor your fluid intake to prevent dehydration and its negative impacts on performance.

Listening to Your Body: Pay attention to how your body responds to different foods and adjust your nutrition plan accordingly. Trust your instincts and intuition.

Making Nutrition a Lifestyle:

Consistency and Moderation: Adopt a sustainable approach to nutrition. Avoid restrictive diets and focus on consistently nourishing your body with wholesome foods.

Mindful Eating: Practice mindful eating to foster a deeper connection with your food and cultivate an awareness of your body's hunger and fullness cues.

Educate Yourself: Stay informed about nutrition trends and developments. Continuously expand your knowledge to make informed choices for your endurance journey.

Balancing Indulgence and Performance:

Occasional Treats: Allow yourself occasional indulgences without guilt. A balanced approach to nutrition includes room for enjoyment and celebration.

Timing Matters: If you indulge, choose the timing strategically. Opt for treats after workouts when your body can better handle the extra calories.

Celebrating Achievements: Use special treats as a way to celebrate milestones and accomplishments along your endurance journey.

Conclusion:

Nutrition is the driving force that propels your strength and endurance towards greatness. By embracing balanced eating, strategic nutrient timing, and a mindful approach to fueling your body, you unleash a powerful source of energy and resilience Remember, nutrition is not just about what you eat but also about the intention and purpose behind it. Embrace nutrition as the key to unlocking your full potential, igniting the fire of strength and endurance that will burn brightly as you journey towards a life of peak performance and optimal well-being.

Chapter 15: Overcoming

Discover strategies for overcoming obstacles and setbacks on your journey. Gain insights into resilience and the power of bouncing back.

Chapter 15: Overcoming - Resilience and the Triumph of Bouncing Back

In the realm of strength and endurance, obstacles and setbacks are inevitable companions on the path to greatness. They test your resolve, challenge your determination, and demand unwavering resilience. In this chapter, we explore the art of overcoming, unveiling strategies to conquer adversity and embrace the power of bouncing back stronger than ever before.

The Essence of Overcoming:

Overcoming is not about avoiding challenges but rather embracing them as catalysts for growth. It is the art of rising above setbacks, harnessing their transformative power, and emerging as a more resilient and determined individual.

Resilience - The Foundation of Endurance:

Embracing the Struggle: Understand that struggle is an integral part of the journey. Embrace it as an opportunity for growth and learning.

Adapting to Change: Resilience lies in your ability to adapt to ever-changing circumstances and continue moving forward.

Positive Self-Talk: Cultivate a positive inner dialogue that empowers you to overcome self-doubt and maintain a strong belief in your abilities.

Strategies for Overcoming Obstacles:

Break It Down: When faced with a daunting challenge, break it down into smaller, manageable tasks. Focus on one step at a time.

Seek Support: Don't hesitate to reach out to your support network —
friends, family, coaches, or mentors — for guidance and encouragement.

Reflect and Learn: After overcoming an obstacle, take time to reflect on
the experience and the lessons it taught you. Use this knowledge to
prepare for future challenges.

The Power of Bouncing Back:

Learn from Failure: Failure is not a dead-end but a stepping stone. Extract
valuable insights from setbacks to improve your approach in the future.

Reshape Your Mindset: Adopt a growth mindset that perceives setbacks
as opportunities for improvement rather than signs of inadequacy.

Resilience in Action: Demonstrate resilience by continuing to pursue your
goals even when faced with setbacks. Your persistence will inspire others
and strengthen your resolve.

Finding Inspiration in Others:

Role Models and Stories: Draw inspiration from the stories of individuals
who have overcome tremendous obstacles to achieve greatness.

Shared Experiences: Connect with fellow endurance enthusiasts who have faced similar challenges. Sharing experiences can provide valuable support and perspective.

Learning from Athletes: Study the experiences of successful athletes and their journeys of overcoming setbacks. Use their strategies as inspiration for your own path.

Embracing the Journey, Not Just the Destination:

Celebrate Progress: Celebrate every step forward, regardless of how small it may seem. Acknowledge the effort and dedication behind each achievement.

Gratitude and Perspective: Practice gratitude for the opportunity to pursue your endurance journey, recognizing that challenges contribute to personal growth.

Embrace Uncertainty: Embrace the uncertainty of the journey. It is through overcoming the unknown that you discover your true strength.

Conclusion:

Overcoming obstacles and setbacks is a testament to your endurance, resilience, and unyielding spirit. Embrace challenges as opportunities to grow and learn, and view setbacks as stepping stones to success. By cultivating a resilient mindset and learning from the experiences of others, you tap into the power of bouncing back stronger and more determined than ever. Remember, the journey of overcoming is a transformative one, shaping you into a person of unwavering strength and fortitude. As you embrace the trials and triumphs, you illuminate the path to greatness, where each obstacle you conquer becomes a testimony to the extraordinary resilience that lies within you.

Chapter 16: Patience

Patience is key in the pursuit of strength and endurance. Understand the importance of gradual progress and the rewards of persistence.

Chapter 16: Patience - The Art of Enduring Progress

In the realm of strength and endurance, patience stands as the virtuous guide, beckoning you to embrace the beauty of gradual progress and the rewards of steadfast persistence. It is the art of waiting with purpose and composure, understanding that the journey to greatness is not a sprint but a marathon. In this chapter, we explore the profound significance of patience in the pursuit of strength and endurance, unveiling the power of enduring progress and the fruits it bears.

The Essence of Patience:

Patience is not passivity but an active state of mind that keeps you anchored to your goals while acknowledging the time and effort required to reach them. It is the art of nurturing resilience, temperance, and the willingness to endure the journey with grace.

The Virtues of Gradual Progress:

Building a Strong Foundation: Patience allows you to build a solid foundation by focusing on fundamental skills and technique before advancing to more complex challenges.

Sustainable Growth: Gradual progress ensures that your body adapts progressively, reducing the risk of injuries and burnout.

Learning and Mastery: Patience allows you to embrace the process of learning and mastery, savoring each milestone as you grow in strength and endurance.

Navigating Plateaus and Setbacks:

Plateaus as Opportunities: Embrace plateaus as periods of consolidation and reflection. They provide opportunities to assess your progress and adjust your approach.

Resilience in Setbacks: Patience enables you to withstand setbacks with resilience, understanding that they are temporary roadblocks on the path to success.

Learning from Challenges: Embrace challenges and setbacks as valuable teachers. They offer insights that foster personal growth and self-discovery.

The Rewards of Steadfast Persistence:

Unveiling Hidden Potential: Patience allows you to unlock hidden potential within yourself, revealing the depths of strength and endurance you didn't know existed.

Emotional Mastery: Steadfast persistence nurtures emotional resilience, helping you maintain focus and composure during difficult times.

The Joy of Progress: Each step forward, no matter how small, becomes a cause for celebration when you recognize the cumulative impact of persistent effort.

Balancing Ambition with Patience:

Setting Realistic Goals: Ambition should be balanced with practicality. Set challenging yet achievable goals to maintain motivation and avoid unnecessary pressure.

Mindful Presence: Stay present in each moment, appreciating the journey rather than solely focusing on the destination.

Trusting the Process: Have faith in the process and believe in the power of consistent effort. Trust that your dedication will yield results in due time.

A Lifelong Journey:

Embracing the Long Haul: Patience is not a fleeting virtue but a lifelong practice. Embrace it as a companion throughout your endurance journey.

Evolving Perspectives: As you progress, your understanding of patience will evolve. Embrace the fluidity of this virtue and adapt your approach accordingly.

Celebrating the Journey: Cultivate gratitude for the opportunity to pursue strength and endurance. Celebrate the progress, the lessons, and the growth that unfolds along the way.

Conclusion:

Patience is the unwavering anchor that steadies your journey to strength and endurance. As you navigate the terrain of gradual progress and persistent effort, you unveil the remarkable rewards that arise from steadfastness. Embrace the art of patience as an integral part of your pursuit, for it is in the embrace of time and resilience that your true potential takes root and flourishes. Remember, the journey of strength and endurance is not just about the destination but the profound transformation that occurs within you. As you cultivate patience, you foster a spirit that transcends momentary triumphs and embodies the enduring greatness that emerges from the heart of patience's unwavering embrace.

Chapter 17: Quality

Focus on quality over quantity in your workouts and daily choices. Learn how prioritizing quality contributes to improved strength and endurance.

Chapter 17: Quality - Elevating Strength and Endurance Through Excellence

In the realm of strength and endurance, the pursuit of excellence rests not in quantity but in the unwavering commitment to quality. It is the art of choosing precision over volume, recognizing that true progress is borne from focused and purposeful actions. In this chapter, we explore the profound significance of prioritizing quality over quantity, unraveling how this mindset elevates strength and endurance to new heights.

The Essence of Quality:

Quality is the heartbeat of excellence. It is the dedication to performing each action with mindfulness, attention to detail, and unwavering commitment.

Mindful Workouts - Embodying Excellence:

Form and Technique: Prioritize correct form and technique in each exercise, ensuring maximum efficiency and reducing the risk of injury.

Focused Intensity: Opt for focused intensity over aimless repetitions. Engage each muscle group with purpose and intention, fostering greater strength gains.

Listening to Your Body: Tune into your body's signals and adjust your workouts accordingly. Quality workouts adapt to your current state of energy and readiness.

The Power of Recovery:

Rest and Rejuvenation: Allow your body ample time to recover and rejuvenate after intense workouts. Quality rests are essential for muscle repair and growth.

Sleep Quality: Prioritize restful sleep to enhance recovery and overall well-being. Quality sleep is a powerful ally in your journey to strength and endurance.

Balancing Intensity: Avoid overtraining by finding the right balance between challenging workouts and giving your body the time it needs to recover.

Nutrition for Nourishment:

Wholesome Choices: Opt for nutrient-dense, whole foods that nourish your body and support optimal performance.

Mindful Eating: Savor each meal with mindfulness, enjoying the flavors and textures, and being conscious of your body's hunger and fullness cues.

Personalized Nutrition: Tailor your nutrition plan to meet your unique needs and goals, seeking guidance from experts if necessary.

Daily Choices, Lasting Impact:

Prioritizing Recovery: Make time for recovery practices such as stretching, meditation, or relaxation techniques to enhance your overall well-being.

Active Lifestyle: Embrace an active lifestyle beyond your workouts, incorporating movement into your daily routines.

Consistency in Excellence: Strive for consistency in your commitment to quality. Each choice you make can have a lasting impact on your strength and endurance journey.

Embracing the Journey of Mastery:

Patience and Progress: Embrace the gradual progress that comes with prioritizing quality. Mastery is a journey that requires time and dedication.

Mindset of Excellence: Cultivate a mindset that celebrates the pursuit of excellence rather than focusing solely on outcomes.

Appreciating the Process: Find joy in the process of refining your skills and pushing the boundaries of your strength and endurance.

Conclusion:

Quality is the beacon that guides you towards excellence in your pursuit of strength and endurance. By prioritizing precision, mindfulness, and purpose in your workouts, nutrition, and daily choices, you elevate your performance and unleash the true potential within you. Embrace each moment as an opportunity to embody excellence, for it is through the commitment to quality that you build a foundation of lasting strength and endurance. Remember, the path to greatness lies not in the quantity of actions but in the mastery of each one. As you walk this path of unwavering commitment to quality, you illuminate the way to a life of strength, endurance, and the pursuit of unyielding excellence.

Chapter 18: R is for Rest - The Restorative Pillar of Endurance

Rest and recovery are essential components of endurance training. Explore the significance of sleep and active recovery in maintaining your overall well-being.

In the realm of strength and endurance, the significance of rest cannot be overstated. It is the restorative pillar that underpins your journey, allowing your body and mind to recover, adapt, and grow. In this chapter, we delve into the profound importance of rest and recovery, exploring the power of sleep and active recovery in maintaining overall well-being on your endurance training odyssey.

The Essence of Rest:

Rest is not a mere pause in your journey but a deliberate act of self-care and rejuvenation. It is the art of giving your body the time and space it needs to heal, restore balance, and prepare for the challenges that lie ahead.

Sleep - The Foundation of Rejuvenation:

Quality Sleep: Prioritize getting enough high-quality sleep each night. Sleep is when your body repairs tissues, consolidates memories, and releases growth hormones.

Sleep Hygiene: Create a conducive sleep environment by minimizing noise, light, and screen time before bedtime.

Consistent Schedule: Establish a consistent sleep schedule to regulate your body's internal clock and improve the quality of your rest.

Active Recovery - Nourishing Movement:

Gentle Exercise: Engage in low-impact, gentle exercises during rest days to promote blood flow, reduce muscle stiffness, and enhance recovery.

Yoga and Stretching: Incorporate yoga or stretching routines into your active recovery to improve flexibility and release tension in muscles.

Mindful Movement: Approach active recovery with mindfulness, being attuned to your body's signals and avoiding pushing yourself too hard.

The Benefits of Rest and Recovery:

Injury Prevention: Proper rest and recovery help prevent overuse injuries and reduce the risk of burnout.

Optimal Performance: Well-rested muscles and a clear mind contribute to improved performance during workouts and endurance challenges.

Mental Clarity: Rest enhances mental clarity and focus, enabling you to make better decisions and adapt to training challenges.

Listening to Your Body:

Recognize Signs of Fatigue: Be mindful of signs of physical and mental fatigue, and adjust your training and rest accordingly.

Respecting Rest Days: Embrace rest days as vital components of your training plan. Avoid the temptation to sk p them in pursuit of more gains.

Recovery as Active Choice: View rest and recovery as active choices rather than passive breaks. Embrace them as opportunities to recharge and emerge stronger.

Holistic Well-Being:

Balancing Life Demands: Prioritize rest ar d recovery to strike a balance between training, work, and personal life.

Mental Well-Being: Rest not only nurtures your physical health but also supports your mental and emotional wel–being.

Self-Care Practices: Embrace self-care practices beyond training, such as meditation or spending time in nature, tc enhance your overall well-being.

Conclusion:

Rest is the restoritive pillar of endurance training, the sacred space where healing and growth take root. By recognizing the significance of sleep and active recovery, you gift yourself the power to endure, excel, and savor the journey. Embrace rest as an essential element of your endurance training, respecting its transformative potential in nurturing both body and mind. As you cultivate the art of rest, you unlock the true essence of endurance, where strength, resilience, and well-being intertwine in a harmonious dance. Remember, the path to greatness is not a relentless pursuit but a balanced rhythm of effort and rest, where each moment of recovery fuels the fire that burns brightly on your endurance journey.

Chapter 19: Self-Care

Prioritize self-care practices that nurture your body, mind, and soul. Discover the connection between self-care and sustained endurance.

Chapter 19: Self-Care - Nurturing the Triad of Endurance

In the tapestry of strength and endurance, the thread of self-care weaves a vital and intricate pattern. It is the art of tending to your body, mind, and soul with unwavering devotion, creating a foundation of holistic well-being that propels you forward on your endurance journey. In this chapter, we delve into the profound significance of self-care, illuminating the profound connection between nurturing yourself and sustaining enduring greatness.

The Essence of Self-Care:

Self-care is not a luxury but a necessity. It is the act of showing up for yourself with love, compassion, and intention, nurturing the triad of body, mind, and soul.

Nurturing Your Body:

Nutritious Fuel: Prioritize nourishing foods that fuel your body for optimal performance and recovery.

Hydration: Maintain proper hydration to support endurance, cognitive function, and overall vitality.

Physical Maintenance: Regularly engage n activities such as foam rolling, massage, and chiropractic care to prevert injuries and promote recovery.

Caring for Your Mind:

Mindfulness Practices: Embrace mindfulness meditation, deep breathing, and visualization to reduce stress and enhance focus.

Stress Management: Identify stress triggers and adopt healthy coping mechanisms, such as journaling, to manage stress effectively.

Positive Self-Talk: Cultivate a positive inner dialogue that empowers you to overcome challenges and embrace a growth mindset.

Nourishing Your Soul:

Time in Nature: Spend time outdoors to rejuvenate your spirit, connect with the natural world, and find solace in its beauty.

Creative Expression: Engage in creative activities that bring you joy, whether it's painting, writing, or playing a musical instrument.

Gratitude Practice: Cultivate a daily practice of gratitude to foster a sense of appreciation and abundance in your life.

The Connection to Sustained Endurance:

Resilience: Self-care nurtures emotional resilience, enabling you to bounce back from setbacks and challenges with renewed strength.

Preventing Burnout: Regular self-care practices help prevent burnout, ensuring you have the energy and enthusiasm to sustain your endurance journey.

Longevity: Prioritizing self-care contributes to your overall health and well-being, supporting longevity in your pursuit of strength and endurance.

Creating a Self-Care Ritual:

Personalized Approach: Tailor your self-care practices to align with your unique preferences, needs, and goals.

Consistency: Make self-care a consistent part of your routine, treating it as an essential appointment with yourself.

Mindful Presence: Approach self-care with mindfulness, fully immersing yourself in the present moment and savoring the experience.

Harmonizing the Triad:

Balance and Harmony: Strive for balance among body, mind, and soul. When all three are nurtured, you create a harmonious foundation for enduring strength.

Interconnectedness: Recognize the interconnectedness of body, mind, and soul. Nurturing one aspect enhances the well-being of the others.

Holistic Greatness: Embrace self-care as the catalyst that propels you toward holistic greatness, where enduring strength flourishes in the embrace of a nurtured and balanced self.

Conclusion:

Self-care is the wellspring from which your endurance journey draws its sustenance. As you prioritize practices that nurture your body, mind, and soul, you forge a path of enduring strength that is both resilient and abundant. Embrace self-care as an essential component of your endurance training, recognizing its transformative power in fostering sustained greatness. As you cultivate the art of self-care, you create a symphony of well-being, where the harmonious interplay of body, mind, and soul elevates your endurance journey to new heights. Remember, the key to enduring strength lies not only in the physical realm but in the holistic embrace of self-care, where each act of nurturing becomes a testament to the enduring greatness that resides within you.

Chapter 20: Technique

Master proper techniques in strength exercises, running, and other activities to optimize performance, prevent injuries, and enhance endurance.

Chapter 20: Technique - The Art of Mastery for Enduring Excellence

In the tapestry of strength and endurance, technique stands as the masterful thread that weaves precision and power into every movement. It is the art of mastering form and execution, guiding you toward optimal performance, injury prevention, and the elevation of endurance. In this chapter, we delve into the profound significance of technique, unveiling how its mastery transforms strength exercises, running, and other activities into avenues of enduring excellence.

The Essence of Technique:

Technique is not a mere mechanical aspect of movement; it is the embodiment of precision, control, and efficiency. It is the gateway to unlocking your true potential and harnessing the energy within each action.

Strength Exercise Mastery:

Form and Alignment: Prioritize proper form and alignment in strength exercises. Maintain a neutral spine, engage the core, and align joints to prevent undue stress.

Mind-Muscle Connection: Cultivate a mind-muscle connection to engage target muscles fully. Focus on the sensation and intention behind each movement.

Progressive Overload: Gradually increase weights and intensity while maintaining proper technique. This ensures steady progress without compromising safety.

Running with Poise:

Footstrike and Posture: Pay attention to your footstrike and posture while running. Land midfoot, lean slightly forward, and engage your core for stability.

Cadence and Stride: Aim for a higher cadence (steps per minute) to reduce impact and improve efficiency. Maintain a comfortable stride length for optimal balance.

Breathing Rhythm: Sync your breathing with your strides to maximize oxygen intake and energy distribution.

Technique Beyond the Gym:

Everyday Movements: Apply proper technique to daily activities such as lifting objects, sitting, and standing. This minimizes strain and promotes posture awareness.

Functional Movements: Optimize technique in functional movements like squatting, bending, and twisting, enhancing overall mobility and joint health.

Mindful Posture: Cultivate mindful posture during work, leisure, and rest to prevent musculoskeletal imbalances and discomfort.

Injury Prevention and Longevity:

Joint Health: Proper technique reduces stress on joints and ligaments, safeguarding them from undue wear and tear.

Muscle Balance: Mastering technique ensures balanced muscle activation, reducing the risk of overuse injuries and muscular imbalances.

Sustained Endurance: By preventing injuries, technique contributes to sustained endurance, allowing you to engage in consistent training and activities.

The Path to Mastery:

Educate Yourself: Seek guidance from experts, trainers, or coaches to learn proper techniques. Invest time in understanding the mechanics of movements.

Mindful Practice: Approach each repetition and movement with mindfulness. Gradually refine your technique through deliberate practice.

Patience and Persistence: Mastery takes time. Embrace the journey of refinement with patience and persistence, celebrating incremental improvements.

Holistic Integration:

Mind-Body Unity: Technique bridges the gap between mind and body, fostering a deeper connection that enhances overall performance and endurance.

Elevating Performance: Proper technique optimizes your energy output, enabling you to perform at your best and endure challenges with greater efficiency.

Enduring Excellence: Technique becomes the cornerstone of your enduring excellence, ensuring that your journey of strength and endurance is grounded in mastery and precision.

Conclusion:

Technique is the art that elevates your journey of strength and endurance from good to exceptional. As you master proper techniques in strength exercises, running, and daily activities, you sculpt a path of precision and power. Embrace technique as an integral part of your training, a compass that guides you toward optimal performance, injury prevention, and the pinnacle of enduring endurance. Remember, the journey of mastery is a dynamic process, and as you refine your techniques, you sculpt a legacy of enduring excellence that stands as a testament to the artistry of movement and the enduring strength within you.

Chapter 21: Unity

Recognize the importance of a supportive community in your journey. Learn how connecting with others enhances your motivation and endurance.

Chapter 21: Unity - The Strength of Community in Endurance

In the vast expanse of strength and endurance, the power of unity shines as a guiding star. It is the force that binds individuals together, creating a supportive and inspiring community that fuels motivation and fortifies endurance. In this chapter, we delve into the profound significance of unity, unraveling the transformative impact of connecting with others on your endurance journey.

The Essence of Unity:

Unity is more than just a shared experience; it is the harmonious symphony of like-minded souls united by a common purpose. It is the recognition that your journey is intertwined with others, and together, you soar to new heights.

The Strength of Support:

Motivation and Accountability: A supportive community provides motivation and accountability, keeping you inspired and on track with your training goals.

Shared Goals: Connecting with others who share similar goals fosters a sense of camaraderie and fuels your determination to push through challenges.

Emotional Resilience: A supportive network provides a safety net during difficult times, helping you navigate setbacks with greater emotional resilience.

The Power of Encouragement:

Positive Reinforcement: Encouraging words and shared successes reinforce your belief in yourself, building confidence in your abilities.

Celebrating Milestones: The community celebrates each other's achievements, creating a collective atmosphere of celebration and pride.

Lifting Each Other Up: During moments of doubt, the community offers a helping hand, lifting you up when you need it the most.

Shared Experiences and Learning:

Wisdom Exchange: Connect with others to share experiences, insights, and knowledge, gaining valuable perspectives and tips for improvement.

Learning Opportunities: Embrace the opportunity to learn from others' successes and challenges, enriching your own endurance journey.

Mentorship and Guidance: Experienced members of the community can offer mentorship and guidance, paving the way for newcomers to succeed.

Finding Your Tribe:

Online Communities: Join virtual platforms, forums, and social media groups focused on strength, endurance, and fitness to find like-minded individuals.

Local Clubs and Events: Explore local clubs and events centered around endurance sports, running, or fitness to connect with individuals who share your passion.

Training Partners: Seek training partners who can accompany you on your workouts, providing companionship and shared goals.

Building a Supportive Culture:

Inclusivity: Create a culture of inclusivity and acceptance within your community, welcoming individuals of all backgrounds and abilities.

Encouraging Positivity: Foster an environment that promotes positivity, uplifting each other and celebrating each person's unique strengths.

Team Spirit: Cultivate a sense of team spirit, where the collective goal is to elevate each member's endurance journey.

Growing Together:

Celebrate Diversity: Embrace the diversity within your community, recognizing that each member brings unique perspectives and experiences.

Evolving Community: As the community grows, adapt to its changing needs, ensuring that it remains a source of support and motivation for all.

Passing the Torch: As you progress in your journey, become a source of support and inspiration for newer members, passing on the torch of unity and endurance.

Conclusion:

Unity is the radiant heart of endurance, where individuals come together to form a mighty force of inspiration and support. As you recognize the importance of a supportive community, you discover the transformative power of connecting with others. Embrace unity as an essential element of your endurance journey, for it is through the strength of community that you soar to new heights of motivation and fortitude. Remember, your journey is not a solitary path, but a collective adventure, where the bonds of unity strengthen your resolve and elevate your endurance to unparalleled greatness.

Chapter 22: Variety

Embrace variety in your workouts and activities to keep things fresh and exciting. Discover the benefits of cross-training and trying new challenges.

Chapter 22: Variety - The Vibrant Tapestry of Endurance

Amidst the landscape of strength and endurance, the vibrant hues of variety paint a mesmerizing masterpiece. It is the palette of diversity that infuses your journey with freshness and excitement, breathing life into your workouts and activities. In this chapter, we delve into the invigorating realm of variety, uncovering the benefits of cross-training and the exhilaration of embracing new challenges.

The Essence of Variety:

Variety is not mere novelty; it is the dynamic force that prevents monotony and rejuvenates your endurance journey. It is the art of infusing different shades of movement into your canvas, creating a vibrant tapestry of experiences.

Elevating Workouts Through Diversity:

Muscle Engagement: Incorporate various exercises to engage different muscle groups, promoting balanced development and reducing the risk of overuse injuries.

Adaptation: Regularly changing exercises and routines prevents your body from plateauing, encouraging continuous adaptation and growth.

Mental Stimulation: Novelty in workouts stimulates your mind, keeping you engaged, focused, and eager to explore new challenges.

The Power of Cross-Training:

Enhanced Conditioning: Cross-training involves diverse activities that improve cardiovascular fitness, muscular endurance, and overall athleticism.

Injury Prevention: Engaging in different forms of exercise reduces the risk of overuse injuries by giving specific muscles and joints time to recover.

Well-Rounded Performance: Cross-training contributes to a well-rounded performance, allowing you to excel in various physical pursuits.

Exploring New Challenges:

Adventure and Excitement: Embrace new challenges, such as obstacle races, hiking, or dance classes, to infuse excitement and adventure into your routine.

Mental Resilience: Conquering unfamiliar challenges builds mental resilience and confidence, enhancing your overall endurance mindset.

Breaking Boundaries: Trying new activities breaks self-imposed limitations, showing you that your endurance extends beyond your comfort zone.

Customizing Variety:

Personal Preferences: Experiment with activities that resonate with your interests and passions, ensuring that variety enhances rather than detracts from your journey.

Periodization: Incorporate variety strategically into your training plan, alternating between different forms of exercise to target specific goals.

Scheduled Exploration: Dedicate specific periods to exploring new activities, allowing yourself to fully immerse and discover hidden strengths.

The Joy of Movement:

Rediscovering Fun: Variety brings an element of playfulness and joy to your workouts, reminding you that movement is a celebration of your body's capabilities.

Sensory Delight: Different activities engage your senses in unique ways, awakening a deeper connection to your physical experience.

Renewed Passion: Variety reignites your passion for movement, reminding you why you embarked on your endurance journey in the first place.

A Lifelong Adventure:

Embrace Change: Embrace the ever-evolving nature of variety, allowing your journey to be an ongoing exploration of movement possibilities.

Cultivating Openness: Approach new challenges and activities with an open heart and mind, ready to learn, adapt, and grow.

Enduring Thrill: Variety becomes the heart's rhythm of your enduring journey, infusing each step with excitement and ensuring that your endurance remains an exhilarating lifelong adventure.

Conclusion:

Variety is the dynamic brushstroke that paints your endurance journey with vibrancy and vitality. As you embrace diversity in your workouts and activities, you breathe new life into your pursuit of strength and endurance. Discover the exhilarating benefits of cross-training and the transformative power of trying new challenges. Embrace variety as an essential facet of your enduring tapestry, where each movement is a stroke of excitement and each challenge an opportunity to grow. Remember, your journey is a canvas of infinite possibilities, where the infusion of variety turns every step into a dance of vibrant endurance.

Chapter 23: Willpower

Cultivate the willpower to stay committed to your fitness goals.
Understand how harnessing your inner strength empowers endurance.

Chapter 23: Willpower - Forging Endurance through Inner Strength

In the realm of strength and endurance, willpower stands as the steadfast
flame that guides you through challenges and fuels your commitment. It is
the inner strength that propels you forward, even when the path seems
arduous. In this chapter, we delve into the profound significance of
willpower, uncovering how harnessing your inner resolve empowers your
journey of endurance.

The Essence of Willpower:

Willpower is not a fleeting emotion; it is the unwavering determination
that fuels your commitment to your fitness goals. It is the force that
propels you to overcome obstacles, persevere through setbacks, and
transform intentions into actions.

The Core of Commitment:

Clear Vision: Cultivate a clear and vivid vision of your fitness goals. This
vision becomes the lighthouse that guides your willpower through storms.

Mindset Mastery: Develop a growth mindset that views challenges as opportunities for growth. This perspective fuels your determination to overcome obstacles.

Resilience: Willpower strengthens your resilience, enabling you to bounce back from setbacks with even greater determination.

Harnessing Inner Strength:

Self-Discipline: Cultivate self-discipline as the cornerstone of willpower. Train yourself to prioritize long-term goals over short-term impulses.

Delayed Gratification: Embrace delayed gratification, understanding that the rewards of enduring effort far surpass the fleeting pleasures of instant gratification.

Emotional Regulation: Develop the ability to regulate your emotions, preventing impulsive decisions driven by momentary feelings.

Powering Through Challenges:

Mental Toughness: Willpower enhances your mental toughness, allowing you to push through discomfort and fatigue during workouts.

Breaking Plateaus: When faced with plateaus or stagnation, willpower helps you persevere and continue working toward progress.

Consistency: Upholding consistent effort even when motivation wanes, showcases the strength of your willpower.

Building a Willpower Arsenal:

Goal Setting: Break your fitness goals into smaller, achievable milestones. Each accomplishment fuels your willpower for the next challenge.

Positive Affirmations: Cultivate positive self-talk and affirmations that reinforce your commitment and remind you of your inner strength.

Visual Cues: Surround yourself with visual cues like quotes, images, or symbols that symbolize your endurance journey and keep your willpower aflame.

Self-Care and Willpower:

Rest and Recovery: Recognize that rest and recovery are crucial for maintaining strong willpower. Burnout weakens your resolve.

Healthy Habits: Nourish your body with balanced nutrition and adequate sleep. Physical well-being fuels mental strength.

Mindfulness Practices: Engage in mindfulness practices such as meditation and deep breathing to keep your mind centered and your willpower focused.

Embodying Enduring Excellence:

The Power of Choice: Willpower reminds you that you have the power to choose your actions and reactions, even in challenging situations.

Legacy of Resilience: Every act of willpower adds a brushstroke to the legacy of your endurance journey—a testament to your strength and commitment.

Sustained Endurance: By cultivating willpower, you ensure that your journey of endurance is not a short-lived endeavor, but a lifelong commitment to health and strength.

Conclusion:

Willpower is the ember that burns within, igniting your endurance journey with unwavering commitment. As you harness your inner strength, you empower yourself to persevere through challenges, cultivate self-discipline, and break through barriers. Embrace willpower as the driving force that propels you toward your fitness goals, transforming your intentions into enduring actions. Remember, your journey of strength and endurance is an ongoing testament to the indomitable willpower within you—a journey that showcases the beauty of forging enduring excellence through the fire of determination.

Chapter 24: Xenial (Hospitality)

Explore the importance of hospitality and supportive relationships in your journey. Learn how kindness and connection contribute to mental and emotional endurance.

Chapter 24: Xenial (Hospitality) - Nurturing Endurance Through Kindness

In the expansive realm of strength and endurance, the art of xenial hospitality emerges as a radiant beacon. It is the warmth of supportive relationships and the power of kindness that infuse your journey with a sense of belonging and elevate your mental and emotional endurance. In this chapter, we delve into the profound significance of xenial hospitality, unveiling how fostering connections and practicing kindness contribute to your enduring well-being.

The Essence of Xenial Hospitality:

Xenial hospitality is not a mere exchange of pleasantries; it is the embodiment of a welcoming heart and open arms. It is the cultivation of supportive relationships that create a nurturing environment, where your endurance journey flourishes.

The Power of Connection:

Community Bonds: Xenial hospitality strengthens the bonds of community, reminding you that you are not alone in your pursuit of strength and endurance.

Emotional Resonance: Supportive relationships provide a safe space to share your struggles and triumphs, fostering emotional resilience and understanding.

Shared Experiences: Connecting with others who share similar journeys fosters a sense of camaraderie and validates your experiences.

Kindness as a Catalyst:

Elevated Mood: Acts of kindness, whether given or received, elevate your mood and contribute to a positive mindset, essential for enduring challenges.

Stress Reduction: Engaging in kind gestures or receiving them releases oxytocin, reducing stress and promoting a sense of well-being.

Mind-Body Harmony: The ripple effect of kindness extends to your physical well-being, creating a harmonious connection between your mind and body.

Supportive Networks:

Family and Friends: Lean on your close-knit circle of family and friends for unwavering support, allowing them to fuel your endurance journey.

Online Communities: Engage with online forums and social media groups dedicated to endurance, finding like-minded individuals who offer advice and encouragement.

Mentorship and Guidance: Seek out mentors who have traversed the path of endurance, benefiting from their wisdom and insights.

Cultivating Kindness:

Self-Compassion: Extend the same kindness to yourself that you offer to others, acknowledging your efforts and celebrating your progress.

Random Acts of Kindness: Infuse your journey with spontaneity by performing random acts of kindness, creating a ripple of positivity around you.

Gratitude Practice: Embrace a daily gratitude practice, focusing on the kindness and support you receive, enhancing your emotional endurance.

Creating a Culture of Hospitality:

Open Arms: Welcome newcomers to the world of endurance with open arms, fostering an inclusive environment that encourages growth.

Positive Encouragement: Offer words of encouragement and celebrate achievements within your community, inspiring each other to endure with a smile.

Empathy and Understanding: Foster empathy and understanding, recognizing that each individual's journey is unique and worthy of respect.

Sustaining Enduring Bonds:

Continual Connection: Nurturing supportive relationships ensures that your endurance journey remains enriched by the kindness of others.

Legacy of Compassion: The kindness you offer and the connections you forge become a lasting legacy, impacting the endurance journeys of generations to come.

Holistic Endurance: Embrace xenial hospitality as a vital pillar of your holistic endurance journey, where the bonds of kindness fortify your mental, emotional, and physical well-being.

Conclusion:

Xenial hospitality is the heart's embrace that elevates your journey of strength and endurance. As you cultivate supportive relationships and practice kindness, you infuse your path with a sense of belonging and emotional well-being. Embrace the power of connection, understanding that your endurance is not a solitary quest but a shared adventure. Remember, your endurance journey is enriched by the generosity of your heart and the bonds of hospitality, creating a legacy of enduring strength and compassion.

Chapter 25: Yoga

Discover the physical and mental benefits of incorporating yoga into your routine. Explore how yoga enhances flexibility, strength, and mental clarity.

Chapter 25: Yoga - The Path to Enduring Balance

In the vast expanse of the endurance journey, the practice of yoga emerges as a sacred pathway toward achieving harmony and well-being. It is a holistic art that weaves together the threads of physical flexibility, strength, and mental clarity. In this chapter, we delve into the profound dimensions of yoga, uncovering how its integration into your routine enhances your endurance, fosters balance, and cultivates lasting well-being.

The Essence of Yoga:

Yoga is not merely a series of poses; it is a transformative journey that unites the body, mind, and spirit. It is the art of conscious movement and breath, inviting you to explore the depths of your physical and mental capabilities.

Physical Flexibility and Strength:

Dynamic Flexibility: Yoga's flowing movements gently stretch and elongate muscles, enhancing flexibility and preventing injuries that can hinder endurance progress.

Muscular Endurance: Holding yoga poses engages and strengthens muscles, promoting overall muscular endurance and balance in your training regimen.

Joint Health: Yoga's emphasis on alignment and controlled movements helps maintain healthy joints, allowing for fluid movement and reducing the risk of strain.

Mind-Body Connection:

Breath Awareness: Yoga places profound importance on breath awareness, teaching you to synchronize your breath with movement. This practice enhances oxygen uptake, supporting your endurance capacity.

Mental Clarity: Through focused breathwork and mindfulness, yoga calms the mind, reducing mental clutter and enhancing your ability to maintain mental clarity during challenges.

Stress Reduction: The meditative aspects of yoga trigger the relaxation response, lowering stress hormones and fostering emotional resilience—a crucial factor in enduring the rigors of training.

Balancing the Endurance Journey:

Recovery and Restoration: Incorporating restorative yoga practices enhances your recovery process, helping to alleviate soreness and promote relaxation after intense workouts.

Preventing Burnout: Yoga's emphasis on mindfulness and balance acts as a counterbalance to the intensity of endurance training, reducing the risk of physical and mental burnout.

Energy Regulation: Yoga's gentle movements and breath control help regulate your energy levels, ensuring you have the vitality needed for consistent endurance efforts.

Customizing Your Yoga Practice:

Classical Yoga: Explore traditional styles like Hatha, Vinyasa, and Ashtanga, each offering unique benefits for your physical and mental endurance.

Yoga Fusion: Blend yoga with other forms of exercise, such as strength training or cardio, to create a balanced cross-training routine.

Restorative Yoga: Integrate restorative practices to rejuvenate your body and mind, facilitating deep relaxation and supporting your endurance recovery.

Embarking on the Yoga Journey:

Mindful Start: Begin your yoga practice mindfully, with an open heart and a willingness to explore the intricacies of movement and breath.

Progressive Approach: Gradually challenge yourself with more advanced poses and sequences, allowing your endurance to evolve in tandem with your yoga practice.

Consistent Commitment: Embrace yoga as an enduring practice, weaving its benefits into your routine to create a seamless tapestry of physical and mental well-being.

Enduring Unity:

Holistic Enrichment: Yoga is a tapestry that weaves together the threads of physical vitality, mental clarity, and spiritual awareness, enhancing your endurance journey's holistic dimension.

Body-Mind Fusion: Through yoga, you foster an enduring unity between your body and mind, allowing them to work harmoniously toward your endurance goals.

A Journey Unveiled: As you tread the path of yoga, you uncover the enduring treasures of balance, flexibility, and mental clarity, unveiling the transformative potential within your endurance journey.

Conclusion:

Yoga is the sacred practice that guides you toward the pinnacle of enduring balance. As you integrate its principles of movement, breath, and mindfulness, you unlock the gateways to physical flexibility, strength, and mental clarity. Embrace yoga as an essential thread woven into the fabric of your endurance journey, enhancing your well-being and empowering your enduring spirit. Remember, your practice of yoga is a dance of unity, a symphony of strength, and a journey of self-discovery that leads to enduring balance and vitality.

Chapter 26: Zeal

Embrace an attitude of enthusiasm and zeal for your journey. Learn how maintaining passion and energy fuels your strength and endurance pursuits.

Chapter 26: Zeal - Igniting the Fire of Enduring Passion

Within the vast landscape of the endurance journey, the spark of zeal illuminates the path with unwavering enthusiasm and energy. It is the boundless passion that fuels your spirit, invigorates your pursuits, and infuses your strength and endurance endeavors with unyielding fervor. In this chapter, we delve into the profound significance of zeal, exploring how its embrace ignites the fire of passion, propelling you toward unwavering strength and enduring vitality.

The Essence of Zeal:

Zeal is not a fleeting emotion; it is the enduring flame that burns within, igniting your journey with boundless enthusiasm and unwavering determination. It is the profound belief in the power of your dreams and the unshakeable commitment to realize them.

Unleashing the Power of Passion:

Fuels Motivation: Zeal is the driving force behind your motivation, pushing you forward when challenges arise and igniting your desire to conquer them.

Enduring Resilience: When passion intertwines with endurance, it gives rise to unyielding resilience, allowing you to persevere through obstacles with unwavering determination.

Sustained Focus: Zeal maintains your focus and dedication, ensuring that your efforts remain directed toward your goals, even amidst distractions.

The Energy of Zeal:

Physical Vitality: Embracing zeal infuses your body with energy, revitalizing your workouts and bolstering your physical endurance.

Mental Alacrity: The fervor of zeal enhances mental clarity and focus, allowing you to make sound decisions and tackle challenges with confidence.

Emotional Fire: Zeal stokes the fire of positive emotions, uplifting your mood and fostering a positive mindset, crucial for enduring the highs and lows of your journey.

Cultivating Zeal:

Align with Purpose: Connect your endurance pursuits with a deeper sense of purpose, anchoring your zeal in meaningful aspirations.

Visualize Success: Envision yourself achieving your goals with passion and enthusiasm, fueling your drive to turn dreams into reality.

Celebrate Progress: Acknowledge and celebrate each milestone on your journey, nurturing your zeal with the joy of accomplishment.

Overcoming Challenges with Zeal:

Mindset of Possibility: Embrace a mindset that sees challenges as opportunities for growth, fueling your zeal to overcome any hurdle.

Adaptability: Zeal empowers you to adapt and find creative solutions when faced with unforeseen obstacles.

Persistence: Zeal ignites your persistence, encouraging you to keep pushing forward, even when the road seems daunting.

Spreading the Fire of Zeal:

Inspiring Others: Let your zeal inspire and uplift those around you, creating a ripple effect of passion within your community.

Encouraging Support: Surround yourself with individuals who share your zeal, offering encouragement and camaraderie on your journey.

Lead by Example: Embody your zeal in action, demonstrating the power of passion and energy to achieve enduring strength and vitality.

Sustaining Enduring Zeal:

Rekindle the Flame: Renew your zeal by revisiting your goals and reminding yourself of the reasons that fuel your passion.

Self-Care: Prioritize self-care to ensure your energy remains replenished, allowing your zeal to burn brightly throughout your journey.

Embrace the Journey: Find joy in the process of endurance, embracing the growth, learning, and transformation it brings.

Conclusion:

Zeal is the unyielding fire that sets your endurance journey ablaze with passion and energy. As you embrace its fervor, you infuse each step with enthusiasm, resilience, and purpose. Let your zeal be the guiding light, illuminating your path toward unwavering strength and enduring vitality. Remember, your journey of passion and energy is an enduring testament to the power of zeal, igniting the fire within to achieve the extraordinary in your life's enduring pursuit.

Conclusion:

"The ABC's of Strength and Endurance" offers a holistic approach to achieving and maintaining physical and mental resilience. By embracing these principles, you can embark on a transformative journey toward a healthier, fitter, and more enduring life. May your commitment, determination, and newfound knowledge lead you to a future of strength and endurance.